Table of Contents

BENEFIT OF ATKINS DIET

1. Weight-Loss: One of the primary benefits of the Atkins Diet is its effectiveness in promoting weight loss. By restricting carbohydrate intake and emphasizing protein and healthy fats, the Atkins Diet can lead to reduced calorie intake and improved fat burning, resulting in significant weight loss for many individuals.

2. Improved Metabolic Health: The Atkins Diet has been shown to improve various markers of metabolic health, including insulin sensitivity, blood sugar control, and lipid profiles. By reducing carbohydrate intake and stabilizing blood sugar levels, the Atkins Diet may help lower insulin levels, reduce inflammation, and decrease the risk of metabolic disorders like type 2 diabetes and metabolic syndrome.

3. Appetite Control: Protein and fat are more satiating than carbohydrates, leading to greater feelings of fullness and reduced hunger on the Atkins Diet. By prioritizing protein-rich foods and healthy fats, individuals may experience improved appetite control and fewer cravings,

making it easier to adhere to the diet and achieve weight loss goals.

4. Increased Energy Levels: Many people report experiencing increased energy levels and improved mental clarity on the Atkins Diet, particularly once they enter a state of ketosis. By relying on fats for fuel instead of carbohydrates, the body can sustain steady energy levels throughout the day, without the fluctuations associated with blood sugar spikes and crashes.

5. Preservation of Lean Muscle Mass: Unlike traditional low-calorie diets, which can lead to muscle loss along with fat loss, the Atkins Diet emphasizes adequate protein intake and resistance training to support muscle preservation. This can help prevent metabolic slowdown and maintain a higher metabolic rate, even during periods of calorie restriction.

6. Favorable Changes in Body Composition: In addition to weight loss, the Atkins Diet may lead to favorable changes in body composition, including reductions in body fat percentage and increases in lean muscle mass. This can result in a more toned and sculpted physique,

along with improvements in overall health and fitness.

7. Flexibility and Personalization: The Atkins Diet offers flexibility in food choices and meal planning, allowing individuals to tailor the diet to their preferences, cultural backgrounds, and dietary needs. With four distinct phases, ranging from strict carbohydrate restriction to gradual reintroduction of carbs, the Atkins Diet can be adapted to accommodate different lifestyles and weight loss goals.

8. Long-Term Sustainability: For many individuals, the Atkins Diet can be a sustainable and lifelong approach to healthy eating and weight management. By promoting whole, nutrient-dense foods and encouraging a balanced macronutrient intake, the Atkins Diet can support long-term adherence and maintenance of weight loss results.

PROS OF ATKINS DIET

1. Effective Weight Loss: The Atkins Diet is renowned for its ability to promote significant and sustainable weight loss. By restricting carbohydrate intake and focusing on protein-rich foods and healthy fats, individuals can achieve a caloric deficit, leading to reduced body fat and improved body composition.

2. Improved Metabolic Health: Research suggests that the Atkins Diet can lead to improvements in various markers of metabolic health, including insulin sensitivity, blood sugar control, and lipid profiles. By stabilizing blood sugar levels and reducing insulin secretion, the diet may lower the risk of metabolic disorders such as type 2 diabetes and metabolic syndrome.

3. Enhanced Appetite Control: High-protein and high-fat foods are inherently more satiating than carbohydrates, leading to increased feelings of fullness and reduced hunger on the Atkins Diet. This can make it easier for individuals to adhere to their dietary goals and manage their calorie intake effectively.

4. Sustainable and Flexible Approach: Unlike many restrictive diets, the Atkins Diet offers flexibility and sustainability, allowing individuals to enjoy a wide variety of foods while still achieving their weight loss and health goals. With four distinct phases that gradually reintroduce carbohydrates, the diet can be adapted to suit individual preferences and lifestyles.

5. Preservation of Lean Muscle Mass: The Atkins Diet prioritizes adequate protein intake and encourages resistance training, which helps preserve lean muscle mass during weight loss. This is important for maintaining metabolic rate and supporting long-term weight management.

6. Favorable Changes in Body Composition: In addition to weight loss, the Atkins Diet often leads to favorable changes in body composition, including reductions in body fat percentage and increases in lean muscle mass. This can result in a more toned and athletic physique, improving overall health and well-being.

7. Improved Energy Levels and Mental Clarity: Many individuals report experiencing increased energy levels and improved mental clarity on the Atkins Diet, particularly once they enter a state of ketosis. By relying on fats for fuel instead of carbohydrates, the body can sustain steady energy levels throughout the day, leading to greater productivity and vitality.

8. Positive Psychological Effects: Successful weight loss and improvements in metabolic health can have significant positive effects on psychological well-being, including increased self-confidence, improved mood, and reduced stress levels. These psychological benefits can further enhance motivation and adherence to the Atkins Diet.

CHICKEN SHAWARMA WITH SWEET POTATOES

Ingredients

2 medium sweet potatoes

1.5 lbs chicken breast tenders

1/4 cup avocado oil or olive oil

1 lemon (juice of)

2 tsp smoked paprika

2 tsp cumin

1 tsp turmeric

1/2 tsp sea salt + more to taste

1/4 tsp cayenne pepper (optional)

1/2 large red onion sliced

fresh parsley or mint for serving (optional)

2 cups arugula (optional)

Instructions

1. Preheat the oven to 425 degrees. Prepare a large sheet pan by gently greasing with cooking spray. Set aside.

2. Peel the sweet potatoes and dice up into even chunks. Place around the outside edges of the pan, and evenly space the potatoes.

3. In a bowl, whisk together oil, lemon, paprika, cumin, turmeric, sea salt, and cayenne pepper if using. Gently brush 1-2 tbsp of the oil mixture over the potatoes. Place the potatoes in the oven. Roast for 15 minutes.

4. Meanwhile, marinate the chicken in the remaining dressing. After 15 minutes, remove the pan from the oven. Place the marinated chicken and red onion in the middle of the sheet pan. Lower the temperature to 400 degrees. Roast for another 20-25 minutes, or until chicken is cooked through.

5. Remove from oven. Serve sweet potatoes, chicken, and onion over arugula (if using), rice, or cauliflower rice. Garnish with parsley or mint. Season with

additional salt and pepper to taste, and additional lemon juice. Or try my tahini dressing.

SHRIMP TACOS

ingredients

For the Taco Marinade:

1/4 cup avocado oil or olive oil

1 lime juiced

1 tbsp tomato paste

1 tbsp coconut aminos

1 tbsp apple cider vinegar

1 clove garlic minced

2 tsp chili powder

1 tsp cumin

1 tsp chipotle powder

1/2 tsp salt

1/4 cup loosely packed cilantro

For the Tacos:

2 lbs raw jumbo shrimp peeled, deveined, and tails removed

1 red bell pepper

1 green bell pepper

1 small red onion thinly sliced

Instructions

1. Preheat the oven to 450 degrees. Line a large baking sheet with foil or lightly grease with a non-stick spray. Set aside.

2. Prepare a quick marinade for the shrimp. Blend in a food processor or blender: oil, juice of 1 lime, tomato paste, coconut aminos, vinegar, chili powder, cumin, chipotle powder, salt, and cilantro. Pour marinade over the shrimp in a bowl while the oven heats up.

3. Line the veggies over the bottom of the sheet pan. Pour shrimp and marinade over the top; spread around the marinade to evenly coat the vegetables.

4. Place in the oven and roast for 8 minutes, then broil for an additional 1-2 minutes or until shrimp is cooked through.

5. Remove from oven. Serve hot over a bed of rice, cauliflower rice, greens, or tortillas

CAULIFLOWER RICE CHICKEN BIRYANI

Ingredients

1 large head of cauliflower

2 tbsp ghee avocado oil, or olive oil

1.5 lbs chicken breast cut into 1 inch pieces

1 medium sized yellow onion diced

2 tbsp finely diced ginger

2 tsp garam masala

1 tsp ground turmeric

3 cloves garlic minced

1 cup diced tomatoes

1/2 cup raisins

1/3-3/4 cup chicken broth

1/2 tsp salt

1/2 cup sliced almonds or chopped

1/4 cup chopped fresh cilantro to taste

Instructions

1. Begin by ricing your cauliflower. Cut your cauliflower into florets. Place inside a high powered blender or food processor and pulse for 10-20 seconds. Scrape down the sides to remove any cauliflower sticking to the side. Once cauliflower is evenly riced, set aside.

2. Heat a large skillet to medium - medium high heat. Add oil or ghee and coat the pan. Toss in chicken and cook for 3-5 minutes, evenly browning all sides (inside might still be a little pink).

3. Now toss in onion and ginger. Stir and cook for another 2-3 minutes.

4. Finally add in spices, salt, tomatoes, chicken broth, and raisins. Mix, then toss in cauliflower rice. Bring mixture to a quick boil, and reduce heat to low. Cover with a lid and let simmer for 5-7 minutes or until cauliflower rice is softened.

5. Remove from heat. Top with almonds and cilantro. Serve hot!

BEEF MEATBALL MINESTRONE SOUP

Ingredients

For the Meatballs

1 lb ground beef or turkey

8 oz pork or turkey sausage

1 tsp dried basil

1 tsp dried oregano

1 tsp garlic powder

1/4 tsp sea salt

For the Soup

2 tbsp olive oil or avocado oil

1 medium white onion diced

2 cloves garlic minced

3 ribs celery diced

2 large carrots peeled and diced

1 medium zucchini diced

1 14 oz can of diced tomatoes

2 tbsp red wine vinegar

5 cups chicken broth

1 tsp sea salt + more to taste

1/4 cup fresh basil chopped

Instructions

For the Meatballs:

1. Heat oven to a broil. In a medium sized bowl, mix together meat with spices. Roll into 1.5 inch balls, and place on a baking sheet. Broil for 4-5 minutes (just enough to get them browned on the outside, they can cook more later). Remove from oven and set aside.

For the Soup:

1. In a large stock pot, heat your pan to medium-medium high heat. Once hot, add diced onion. Cook for 3-4 minutes.

2. Now add garlic, celery, zucchini, and carrots. Cook for another 2-3 minutes, then add tomatoes, broth, and vinegar. Bring to a boil, then add meatballs to soup.

3. Reduce heat to a simmer, let cook uncovered for about 20 minutes. Season with salt.

4. Top with fresh basil to serve and parmesan cheese (optional)

POT EGG ROLL IN A BOWL

Ingredients

1 tbsp avocado oil or olive oil

1 lb ground beef, turkey or pork

3 tsp chopped fresh ginger

2 cloves garlic minced

1/3 cup coconut aminos

1/3 cup beef broth

1/4 cup rice vinegar

1 tbsp sesame oil

4 cups shredded cabbage divided

2 cups shredded carrots divided

1/4 cup chopped fresh cilantro optional

3 tbsp chopped green onion optional

3 tbsp hot sauce optional

4 cups cauliflower rice for serving

Instructions

1. Select the saute function on the Instant Pot. Once hot, coat the bottom of the pot with oil. Add the meat and begin to brown. After 3-4 minutes, add in the ginger and garlic. Cook for another 2-3 minutes, or until meat is no longer pink. Select cancel.

2. Meanwhile make the sauce. In a bowl, mix together coconut aminos, broth, rice vinegar, and sesame oil. Pour on top of the meat mixture and deglaze the pan, ensuring nothing is stuck at the bottom.

3. Place 3 cups of cabbage, + 1 cup carrots on top of the meat mixture. Secure the lid. Select manual and cook on high pressure for 5 minutes. Once cook time is complete, release all steam.

4. Top mixture with remaining cabbage and carrots. Serve over cauliflower rice. Add onion, cilantro, and hot sauce if using.

ORANGE CHICKEN AND BROCCOLI

Ingredients

1.5 lbs chicken cut into bite sized pieces

1.5 tbsp arrowroot starch*

1/2 cup coconut aminos or GF Tamari Soy Sauce

1/3 cup fresh squeezed orange juice

2 tsp orange zest

1/4 cup rice vinegar

2 tsp sesame oil

3 cloves crushed garlic divided

3 tsp finely chopped ginger divided

1 tsp crushed red pepper optional

3 cups chopped broccoli

2 tsp sesame seeds optional

2 tbsp chopped green onion optional

Instructions

1. In a small bowl, whisk together the sauce ingredients: coconut aminos, orange juice, vinegar, sesame oil, orange zest, 2 cloves crushed garlic, 2 tsp fresh ginger, and crushed red pepper (if using).

2. Place chicken and arrowroot starch inside a resalable bag or container. Shake around until chicken is well coated.

3. Select the saute function on your Instant Pot. Once hot, add the avocado oil, 1 tsp garlic, and 1 tsp chopped ginger. Stir, then add chicken. Cook for 1-2 minutes until the chicken is slightly browned. Select the cancel function.

4. Now pour the sauce on top of the chicken. Secure the lid, ensuring the valve is in the sealed position. Select "manual" or "pressure" function and cook on high pressure for 7 minutes.

5. Once cooking is complete, use a quick release. Remove the lid once the steam has been released, and toss in chopped broccoli. Stir, and place the lid back on the IP to let the broccoli steam and cook for another 3 to 4 minutes.

6. Serve over rice or cauliflower rice with sesame seeds and green onion (if using).

7. For slow cooker, follow the same instructions with the whisking of the sauce. Coat the chicken with arrowroot starch like above and place chicken inside your slow cooker. Pour sauce over the top. Cook on low for 4-5 hours.

BEEF STROGANOFF

Ingredients

1.5 lbs sirloin steak tips or lean stew beef cut into small pieces

1/2 large white onion chopped

3 cloves garlic minced

10 oz sliced mushrooms

1 1/4 cup beef broth

1/4 cup coconut aminos or GF tamari soy sauce

1/4 cup red wine vinegar

1/2 tsp onion powder

1/2 tsp garlic powder

1/2 cup canned coconut milk or coconut cream

3 tbsp arrowroot starch

2 tbsp water

Salt and pepper to taste

Instructions

For the Slow Cooker

1. Place beef inside your slow cooker, and top with onions, mushrooms, and garlic.

2. In a separate bowl, mix together broth, soy sauce, vinegar, onion powder, and garlic powder. Pour on top of beef and vegetables.

3. Set your slow cooker to low and cook for 5 hours.

4. At the five hour mark, add coconut cream.

5. In a separate small bowl, mix together arrowroot starch and water. Add to slow cooker.

6. Let simmer for another 30 mins – 1 hour or until sauce is thickened and beef is tender.

7. Serve over cauliflower rice, or rice.

For the Instant Pot:

1. Select the saute function on your instant pot. Once hot, add about 1 tbsp olive oil or avocado oil to coat the bottom of your pan. Saute onions for about 2 minutes, then add garlic and cook for another 1-2 minutes. Select cancel.

2. Season your beef with garlic & onion powder, and a bit of salt and pepper. Place on top of the onion/garlic mixture.

3. In a small bowl, mix together broth, coconut aminos, and vinegar. Pour on top of the meat. Add mushrooms.

4. Secure the lid to your Instant Pot. Cook on high pressure for 15 minutes. Use a natural release. After opening the lid, add in coconut milk or cream and stir.

If it needs more heat to dissolve, select the saute function.

5. Stir in arrowroot starch and water to thicken.

6. Serve over cauliflower rice or zoodles.

GREEK CHICKEN

Ingredients

2 tbsp olive oil or avocado oil

3 cloves garlic

2 lbs chicken thighs boneless, skinless

1/2 tsp salt

1/4 tsp pepper (can use lemon pepper)

1 12 oz jar marinated roasted red peppers drained and diced

1 8 oz jar marinated artichoke hearts drained

1 cup kalamata olives

1/2 medium red onion sliced

2/3 cup chicken broth

1/4 cup red wine vinegar

1/2 lemon juiced

1 tsp dried oregano

1 tsp dried thyme

1-2 tbsp arrowroot starch

tbsp fresh basil chopped

1/2 cup crumbled feta optional

Instructions

For the Slow Cooker:

1. Begin by heating a skillet to medium high heat. While skillet is heating, salt and pepper each side of your chicken thighs. Add oil to the hot skillet, then crushed garlic. Cook for 1 minute, now add chicken. Sear chicken on each side for about 2 minutes (no need to cook all the way through).

2. Place chicken on the bottom of your slow cooker. Now arrange the artichoke hearts, peppers, and olives around the chicken filling in the gaps on the bottom of your slow cooker. Top with sliced red onion.

3. In a bowl, mix together 1/2 cup of chicken broth (don't need the full 2/3 for slow cooker), vinegar, lemon, dried oregano, and dried thyme. Pour on top of the chicken/vegetable mixture. Place lid on top.

4. Cover and cook for 4 hours on low or 2-3 hours on high. Remove lid.

5. Spoon out some of the juice into a small bowl once cooking is complete. Add 1 tbsp of arrowroot starch to the juice, whisk, and pour back into the slow cooker. Allow the sauce to thicken for another 15-20 minutes before serving.

6. Serve over potatoes, rice, or cauliflower rice. Top with fresh herbs, sprinkle with additional salt and pepper, and optional feta.

For the Instant Pot:

1. Select the saute function on your Instant Pot. While pot is heating, salt and pepper each side of your chicken thighs. Add oil to the hot pot, then crushed

garlic. Cook for 1 minute, now add chicken. Sear chicken on each side for about 2 minutes (no need to cook all the way through).

2. Now arrange the artichoke hearts, peppers, and olives around the chicken filling in the gaps on the bottom of your Instant Pot (if there are any). It's okay to let some of those veggies sit on top of the chicken. Top with sliced red onion.

3. In a bowl, mix together chicken broth, vinegar, lemon, dried oregano, and dried thyme. Pour on top of the chicken/vegetable mixture. Secure the lid.

4. Select the manual function (this may also be called "pressure" on certain versions of Instant Pot). Adjust the time using +- button to 7 minutes (this will cook on high pressure for 7 minutes).

5. Once cooking is complete, use a quick release (natural release is also fine). Be sure to turn your valve down and release all steam before opening the lid.

6. Spoon out some of the juice into a small bowl once cooking is complete. Add 2 tbsp of arrowroot starch to the juice, whisk, and pour back into the Instant Pot. Allow the sauce to thicken for a few minutes before serving.

7. Serve over potatoes, rice, or cauliflower rice. Top with fresh herbs, sprinkle with additional salt and pepper, and optional feta.

FLAKY LEMON PEPPER SALMON

Ingredients

¾ cup water

A few sprigs of parsley, dill, tarragon, basil or a combo

1.5 lb salmon filet skin on

2 tbsp ghee or other healthy fat divided

¼ tsp salt or to taste

½ tsp pepper or to taste

1/2 lemon thinly sliced + more to taste

1 zucchini julienned

1 red bell pepper julienned

2 carrots julienned

Instructions

1. Place water and herbs in the Instant Pot and then put in the steamer rack making sure the handles are extended up.

2. Drizzle salmon with 1 tbsp ghee/fat, season with salt and pepper, and cover with lemon slices. Place salmon, skin down on rack.

3. Close the Instant Pot and make sure the vent is sealed. Select the "Steam" function (you can also use manual/high pressure) and press the + or − buttons to set it to 3 minutes.

4. While salmon cooks, julienne your veggies.

5. When cooking is complete, use a quick release. Select the cancel button. Remove lid, and using hot pads, carefully remove rack with salmon and set on a plate.

6. Remove herbs and discard. Add veggies and select the "Sauté" function and let the veggies cook for

another 2 to 3 minutes using the residual butter/ghee and lemon juice.

7. Serve salmon with veggies on top. Add remaining tbsp of butter/ghee to the pot and pour a little of the sauce over veggies and salmon if desired. Top with any additional fresh herbs and a squeeze of lemon juice.

SAUSAGE, KALE, AND SWEET POTATO SOUP

Ingredients

2 tbsp olive oil

1 lb ground turkey or pork sausage

1 medium white onion chopped

3 cloves garlic minced

2 large sweet potatoes skinned and chopped

10 oz sliced mushrooms

5 cups chicken broth

1 cup dry white wine*

2 tbsp apple cider vinegar

1 tbsp dried basil

1 tsp sea salt plus extra to taste

1/2 tsp fresh ground pepper

3 cups roughly chopped kale

2 tbsp freshly chopped thyme optional

Instructions

1. For the Instant Pot:

2. Select the saute function on your instant pot. Let it heat up (about 2 minutes). Add olive oil to coat the pot, and toss in ground sausage. Cook until almost cooked through, about 5 minutes. Add onion and garlic. Cook for another 3-4 minutes.

3. Add sweet potatoes, mushrooms, chicken broth, wine, vinegar, dried basil, salt, and pepper. Secure the lid.

4. Select manual and cook at high pressure for 8 minutes. Select cancel and use a quick release.

5. Open lid and add kale. Let cook with lid open for another 3-4 minutes, or until kale is softened but not wilted. Add additional salt if needed. Garnish with fresh thyme and serve.

6. For the Slow Cooker:

7. Heat up a large skillet to medium high heat. Coat your pan with olive oil and add sausage. Cook for 5 minutes, then add in onion and garlic and cook another 3-4 minutes.

8. Place sausage mixture in your slow cooker. Add sweet potatoes, mushrooms, chicken broth, white wine, vinegar, basil, salt, and pepper.

9. Set your slow cooker to low and cook for 4 hours.

10. At the end of 4 hours, add kale and stir. Let cook for another 10-15 minutes, or until kale has softened.

11. Serve hot with fresh thyme.

CARNITAS

Ingredients

3-4 lbs Pork shoulder fat trimmed and cut into 4 pieces

1 tbsp avocado oil or olive oil

2 tsp chili powder

2 tsp cumin

1 tsp oregano

1/2 tsp sea salt + extra for taste

2-3 large oranges juice of

2 limes juice of

1 yellow onion quartered

3 cloves garlic

cilantro for garnish

Instructions

1. Select the saute function on the Instant Pot. Once hot, coat with oil. Place the 4 pieces of pork in the IP, and saute on all sides until lightly browned (less than 8 minutes total). Remove the pork, set aside. Select cancel.

2. De-glaze the pan with the juice from the oranges and limes. In a small bowl, combine the spices. Combine with the orange/lime juice inside the IP. Place the pork inside, then top with onion and garlic. Secure the lid. Set your oven to broil (optional)

3. Cook on high pressure (manual) for 25 minutes. Use a quick release. Remove the pork and shred with a fork. Place on a baking sheet and add to oven. Broil for 4-5 minutes (optional, but such a great step to finish off).

4. Serve hot and spoon additional sauce from the IP on top of the pork. You can wrap in tortillas, serve in a bowl of greens, serve over rice, or serve over cauliflower rice. Garnish with cilantro and any other additional toppings you enjoy.

LEMON CHICKEN AND ASPARAGUS SOUP WITH BASIL

Ingredients

1 lb chicken breast or tenders

3 tbsp avocado or olive oil divided

3 cloves garlic crushed

8 large asparagus stalks

2 14 oz cans full fat coconut milk

2-3 cups chicken broth

Juice of 1 lemon about 1/4 cup

1 tbsp lemon zest

Salt and Pepper to taste

1/4 cup chopped fresh basil

Instructions

1. To prep this dish: chop your chicken breast or tenders into 1 inch chunks. Season with a bit of salt and pepper.

2. Heat a large soup pot to medium high heat, once hot add in 1 tbsp avocado or olive oil. Add chicken to the pot, and cook for about 3-4 minutes until all sides are lightly golden (chicken may be undercooked inside). Set aside.

3. While chicken is cooking, prepare your asparagus. Chop about 1/2 inch off each end. Slice the remaining stalk in 1 inch pieces.

4. Add in another tbsp oil to the soup pot, toss in garlic and asparagus. Cook for 8-10 minutes or until asparagus is crispy. Toss chicken back into the pot.

5. Add coconut milk and 2 cups broth to the pot. Check to see level of liquid, if you prefer a more liquid soup, add in an additional 1/2-1 cup broth. Heat to a soft boil, then reduce to low. Let simmer for 5-7 minutes, stirring frequently and letting flavors meld.

6. Just before serving, add lemon juice and lemon zest to the pot. Season with salt and pepper.

7. Place soup in individual bowls, garnish with fresh basil.

Paprika Smashed Potatoes

Ingredients

16 ounces baby gold potatoes, about 12 - 16 depending on the size

kosher salt

3/4 teaspoon sweet paprika

1/2 teaspoon freshly ground black pepper

1/4 teaspoon garlic powder

1 teaspoon extra virgin olive oil

Reynolds wrap heavy duty foil

chopped parsley, for garnish

Instructions

Place the potatoes in a medium pot and cover with cold water, add 1 teaspoon kosher salt. Bring to a boil and cook until a knife easily pierces to the center of each potato, about 18 - 20 minutes. Remove from water and dry, place on a clean work surface and gently press using the bottom of a glass to smash the potato.

Preheat the oven to 425F. Line a sheet pan with foil.

In a small bowl combine paprika, 1/2 teaspoon salt, black pepper and garlic powder. Place potatoes in a single layer on the prepared sheet pan. Lightly brush potatoes with oil and sprinkle both sides of each potato with spice mix.

spices

Bake 20 minutes, turning halfway until crisp and golden. Garnish with parsley.

Garlic Shrimp

Ingredients

1 1/4 lbs large shrimp, peeled and deveined (weight after you peel them)

6 cloves garlic, sliced thin

1 1/2 tbsp extra virgin Spanish olive oil, or any good quality olive oil

crushed red pepper flakes, to taste

1/4 teaspoon sweet Spanish paprika, or more to taste

pinch kosher salt

1/4 cup parsley, chopped

Instructions

In a large skillet, heat oil on medium heat and add the garlic and red pepper flakes.

In a large skillet, heat oil on medium heat and add the garlic and red pepper flakes.

Sauté until golden, about 2 minutes being careful not to burn.

Add shrimp and season with a pinch of salt and paprika.

Cook 2-3 minutes until shrimp is cooked through. Do not overcook or it will become tough and chewy. Add chopped fresh parsley and divide equally in 4 plates.

Coconut Red Curry Shrimp Skewers

Ingredients

1 ½ lbs large, 20-25 shrimp, peeled

½ tsp kosher salt

1 red onion

½ cup low-fat coconut milk

2 Tbsp red curry paste, or more to taste

1 ½ tsp minced or grated fresh ginger

2 cloves garlic, minced or grated

½ jalapeño, minced (optional)

2 limes

2 red bell pepper

8 or 16 large skewers

Cooking spray

Chopped cilantro for serving

Instructions

Pat the shrimp dry and season both sides with salt.

Cut the onion into 8 wedges and reserve 7 wedges for the skewers.

Mince the remaining wedge and add it to a large bowl with the coconut milk, curry paste, ginger, garlic, and jalapeño (if using) along with the zest and juice of 1 lime.

Whisk until smooth, then give it a taste; if you'd like a stronger curry flavor, add a little more paste.

Red Curry Marinade

Add the shrimp to the bowl and marinate for 30 minutes.

Meanwhile, preheat the grill with high heat and oil the grates.

Cut the reserved onion wedges into approximately 1-inch chunks, and try to keep the layers intact.

Cut the bell pepper into 1- to 2-inch pieces.

Thread the shrimp, onion wedges, and [individual or doubled slices of] bell pepper onto doubled skewers, alternating as you like but beginning and ending each skewer with shrimp, for a total of 8 kabobs.

Reserve the marinade and lightly spray the kabobs with cooking oil.

Add the kabobs to the grill and brush with marinade. Grill for 2 to 3 minutes per side, brushing with marinade after flipping, until the shrimp are pink and firm and the onion is lightly charred.

To serve, place the kabobs on a platter. Generously sprinkle chopped cilantro over everything and serve with wedges of lime.

Grilled Steak With Tomatoes, Red Onion And Balsamic

Ingredients

2 lb flank or london broil steak

1 1/2 teaspoons kosher salt and fresh black pepper, to taste

garlic powder

1 tbsp extra virgin olive oil

2 tbsp balsamic vinegar

1/3 cup red onion, chopped

3 to 4 medium tomatoes, chopped (about 3 1/2 cups)

1 tbsp fresh herbs such as oregano, basil or parsley

Instructions

Pierce steak all over with a fork. Season generously with salt, pepper and garlic powder and set aside about 10 minutes at room temperature.

In a large bowl, combine onions, olive oil, balsamic, salt and pepper. Let onions sit a few minutes in the mixture to mellow a bit. Combine with tomatoes and fresh herbs and adjust seasoning if needed.

Heat grill or broiler on high heat. Cook steak about 7 minutes on each side for medium rare or longer to taste. Remove from grill and let it rest on a plate for about 5 minutes before slicing.

Slice steak thin on the diagonal; top with tomatoes and serve.

Grilled Bruschetta Chicken

Ingredients

3 medium vine ripe tomatoes

2 small cloves garlic, minced

1/4 cup chopped red onion

2 tbsp fresh basil leaves, chopped

1 tbsp extra virgin oil

1 tbsp balsamic vinegar

kosher salt and fresh cracked pepper to taste

3 oz part skim mozzarella, diced (omit for whole30, paleo)

1.25 lbs 8 thin sliced chicken cutlets

Instructions

Combine onion, olive oil, balsamic, 1/4 tsp kosher salt and pepper. Set aside a few minutes.

Chop tomatoes and place in a large bowl. Combine with garlic, basil, onion-balsamic combo and additional 1/8 tsp salt and pepper to taste. Set aside and let it sit at least 10 minutes or as long as overnight.

Toss in the cheese when ready to serve.

Season chicken with salt and fresh pepper.

Preheat the grill to medium-high, clean and oil the grates to prevent sticking.

Grill the chicken 2 minutes on each side, set aside on a platter and top with bruschetta and serve.

Shrimp Ceviche

Ingredients

1 pound fresh peeled and deveined shrimp, chopped (preferably wild)

1 cup fresh squeezed lime juice, from 6 to 9 limes

1/4 cup chopped red onion

1 1/2 teaspoons kosher salt

2/3 cup peeled and diced cucumber

1 to 2 jalapeño, stemmed and sliced into rings

1/4 cup chopped cilantro

1 scallions, chopped

tortilla chips or plantain chips, for serving

Instructions

In a large bowl combine the shrimp, lime juice, red onion and salt.

How To Make Ceviche

Let it sit for 20 minutes, stirring occasionally until opaque.

Add the cucumbers, jalapeño, cilantro and scallion.

Easy Ceviche Recipe With Shrimp

Serve right away with chips.

Pico De Gallo Salsa

Ingredients

4 medium ripe tomatoes, chopped

1/2 cup finely chopped white onion

1-2 jalapeño or serrano pepper, seeded and finely chopped

1/4 cup finely chopped fresh cilantro leaves, no stems

2 tbsp fresh lime juice

kosher salt and pepper, to taste

2 tbsp chopped red bell pepper, (optional)

1 clove garlic, minced (optional)

Instructions

In a bowl combine all ingredients.

Let it marinate in the refrigerator at least an hour for best results.

Low-Yolk Egg Salad

Ingredients

4 large hard boiled eggs, peeled

4 teaspoons light mayonnaise, *check labels for whole30

1/2 teaspoon Dijon mustard

2 tbsp chopped green scallions or chives

kosher salt and fresh pepper to taste

Instructions

Separate the yolks from the egg whites and discard 2 of the yolks. (My dog loves them!)

Half Yolk Egg Salad

Chop the eggs and combine with mayonnaise, dijon mustard, scallions, salt and pepper.

Turkey Picadillo

Ingredients

1.33 lb 93% lean ground turkey

4 oz tomato sauce, (1/2 can)

1 tsp kosher salt

1 tsp ground cumin

2 small bay leaves

2 tbsp green Spanish pitted olives, plus 2 tbsp brine

Sofrito:

1 medium tomato

1/2 medium onion, finely chopped

2 cloves minced garlic

2 tbsp red bell pepper, finely chopped

2 tbsp cilantro, optional

Instructions

Brown the ground turkey on medium heat in large sauté pan and season with salt and pepper. Use a wooden spoon to break the meat up into small pieces.

cooking ground turkey

Meanwhile, while turkey is cooking, make the sofrito by chopping onion, garlic, pepper, tomato and cilantro. (I quickly do it in my mini chopper)

Add sofrito to the meat and continue cooking on a low heat.

Add olives and about 2 tbsp of the brine (this adds great flavor) cumin, bay leaves, and more salt if needed.

Add tomato sauce and 1/4 cup of water and mix well.

Reduce heat to low and simmer covered about 15 to 20 minutes to let the flavors meld.

Spanakopita Baked Eggs

Ingredients

1-1/2 lbs frozen spinach, thawed [24 ounces]

1 tsp olive oil

1/2 medium yellow onion, thinly sliced [1 1/2 cups]

1 tsp kosher salt

1/2 cup chopped scallions, [3-5 scallions depending on the size]

1/2 cup chopped dill

3/4 cup crumbled feta

Juice of 1 lemon

Black pepper, to taste

4 large eggs

Instructions

Preheat the oven to 375F degrees.

Squeeze most of the water out of the spinach, but you don't have to go crazy—a little water left is fine and will cook off in the oven.

Heat a large ovenproof skillet over medium-high heat. When hot, add 1 tsp olive oil, then add the onion and

1/2 tsp salt, and cook until tender and translucent, 3 to 5 minutes.

Add the scallions and cook, stirring constantly, until just starting to soften, about 1 minute.

Add the spinach, dill, 1/2 cup feta, lemon juice, remaining 1/2 tsp salt, and pepper and mix until everything is well-combined and heated through. Remove from the heat.

Make four wells in the top, crack an egg into each, and season each with a little salt and pepper.

Top spinach with remaining 1/4 cup Feta.

Carefully transfer the skillet to the middle rack and bake just until the egg whites are set, 8 to 13 minutes, to your desired liking.

Hearts Of Palm Noodle Peanut Stir Fry

Ingredients

1 tbsp sesame oil, divided

1 clove garlic, minced

1 -1/2 teaspoons fresh ginger

1 12 ounce package Palmini (hearts of palm) linguini

1 tbsp low sodium soy sauce, or liquid aminos for whole30

1 teaspoon sriracha

1-1/2 cups baby spinach

1 tablespoon peanut butter, or almond butter for whole30

1 large egg

sesame seeds, for topping

scallions, for garnish

Instructions

In a large nonstick skillet heat 1/2 tablespoon oil, add the garlic and ginger and cook until fragrant, 30 seconds.

Add the hearts of palm noodles and stir.

Add 1 tbsp soy sauce, sriracha, and stir cook 1 minute, add spinach and cook until wilted, 2 to 3 minutes then push to one side.

Add peanut butter on the other side and leave until melted, about 30 seconds then mix all together.

Push everything to the side.

Add remaining oil on the other side and crack the egg, scramble then mix all together.

Transfer to a bowl, top with more sriracha, sesame seeds and scallions.

Harissa Chicken Meatballs

Ingredients

1 pound ground chicken

1 teaspoon kosher salt

1/2 teaspoon smoked paprika

1/2 cup frozen riced cauliflower

1/4 cup chopped onion

1/4 cup packed chopped parsley

3 large peeled garlic cloves, minced

1 large egg

Olive-oil cooking spray

2 jars, 10 oz each prepared mild harissa sauce (I love Mina Harissa)

Instructions

Place chicken in a large mixing bowl, break- up slightly. Sprinkle with 1 teaspoon salt and smoked paprika.

Add frozen cauliflower, parsley, onion, garlic, and egg and mix just until ingredients are combined. Avoid over-mixing. Divide chicken mixture into 16 portions (about 1 1/4 ounce each); gently shape into balls.

Heat a heavy-duty non-stick large skillet (with tall sides) over medium-high heat.

Spray with olive oil cooking spray, add meatballs and cook, turning occasionally to brown on all sides, about 6 minutes.

Pour in harissa and allow mixture to reach a simmer, reduce heat to medium-low and continue to simmer for 20 to 25 minutes.

Avocado Salsa

Ingredients

6 roma tomatoes, seeded and diced

1/2 red onion, chopped

1 jalapeno, seeded and chopped

4 avocados, peeled, cored, and diced

2 limes, juiced

1/2 teaspoon salt

1/2 cup cilantro leaves, chopped

Instructions

In a large bowl, combine all of the ingredients. Give everything a toss and taste test to see if you need additional salt.

Serve and enjoy.

Best Salsa(Easy Restaurant-Style)

Ingreidents

2 cloves garlic

1/2 yellow onion, roughly chopped

1 jalapeno pepper, seeded and roughly chopped

2 14-ounce cans fire-roasted diced tomatoes, drained

1 4-ounce can green chilies

1/2 cup fresh cilantro, approx 1/2 a bunch

1/2 lime , juiced

1/2 teaspoon salt, to taste

Instructions

Add the onion, garlic and jalapeno to the food processor first. These ingredients will be chopped finer if they're on the bottom.

Then add the drained tomatoes, green chilies (no need to drain), cilantro, lime juice and salt.

Pulse in one second increments. Keep pulsing until the salsa is well-blended, but still a little chunky.

Season to taste with additional salt, or lime juice, if needed.

Serve the salsa immediately or store it for later.

Vegan Tzatziki

Ingredients

1 cup raw cashews, soaked 4-6 hours (or overnight)

1/2 cup water

1/4 cup fresh lemon juice

1/2 medium cucumber, peeled and shredded

1 clove garlic

2 tablespoon fresh dill, chopped

1/2 teaspoon sea salt

Instructions

Soak your cashews overnight. Then drain and thoroughly rinse them.

Blend the cashews, water, lemon juice and garlic in a high-powered blender for 1-2 minutes, or until creamy.

Place the shredded cucumber in a fine mesh sieve over a bowl and press down to remove excess liquid. Alternatively, you could use a nut milk bag to sqeeze out the liquid.

Pour the cashew mixture into a mixing bowl. Add the drained cucumber, dill and salt, then stir together to combine.

Chill for 30 minutes before serving.

Mango Salsa

Ingredients

2 ripe mangos, peeled, pitted, and diced

1/2 small red onion, diced

1 medium cucumber, sliced and diced

1 jalapeno, seeded and finely diced

1/2 cup cilantro leaves, finely chopped

1 lime, juiced

1/4 teaspoon salt

Instructions

Once you have prepared all the ingredients, toss them into a bowl and stir everything together until it's combined.

Bacon Deviled Eggs - Deviled Eggs With Bacon

Ingredinets

6 hard boiled eggs, cooled and peeled

3 tablespoon mayonnaise

1 tablespoon pickle relish

1 teaspoon Dijon mustard

salt and pepper, to taste

2 slices bacon, cooked and crumbled

1 tablespoon chives, finely diced

Instructions

Slice the hard boiled eggs in half lengthwise. Remove the yolk to a small bowl with a spoon and place the egg whites on a plate.

Mash the yolks with a fork and add the mayonnaise, pickle relish, mustard, salt and pepper. Stir everything together until it's creamy.

Use a spoon to add a portion of the deviled egg mixture back into the hole of each egg white.

Garnish with a generous amount of bacon bits and top with a sprinkle of chives.

Avocado Deviled Eggs

Ingredients

6 hard-boiled eggs

1 avocado, peeled and pitted

1 lime, juiced

2 tbsp red onion, finely chopped

2 tbsp cilantro, finely chopped

1 tsp garlic powder

salt and pepper, to taste

Instructions

Cut the hard boiled eggs in half and scoop out the yellow egg yoke to a mixing bowl. Place the hard boiled egg white halves on a serving platter.

To the mixing bowl of egg yolks, add the avocado, lime juice, red onion, cilantro, garlic powder, salt and pepper.

Use a fork and mash all of the ingredients together until nice and creamy.

Scoop the mixture with a spoon and dollop it back into the egg white halves. Alternatively, you could use a piping bag to pipe the avocado egg mixture into the egg white halves.

Garnish with extra red onion and cilantro, then serve and enjoy!

CONCLUSION

The Atkins Diet represents a valuable tool in the arsenal of weight loss and metabolic management strategies, offering a scientifically sound and practical approach to achieving sustainable health and well-being.With its focus on whole foods, balanced nutrition, and individualized support, the Atkins Diet continues to hold promise as a viable solution for those seeking lasting results in their quest for optimal healt